MW01147570

Essential Oils for Rapid Weight Loss

The Complete Guide to Losing Weight
Fast Using Essential Oils

by FlatBelly Queens

Published in Great Britain by:

FlatBelly Queens
345 Old Street
London
EC1V 9LE

© Copyright 2016 – Flatbelly Queens

ISBN-13:978-1536905274
ISBN-10:1536905275

Table of Contents

INTRODUCTION:

You have been looking for a new and effective way to lose weight and have struggled with doing so. Dieting and depriving yourself is making you irritable and frustrated, especially since nothing else seems to work. You need a new and effective way to lose weight

The answer you are looking for is here in this book. Using essential oils for weight loss is a time-honored tradition, something that you can easily incorporate into your life, and a proven way to make dieting and losing weight easier for you. Essential oils can do a great many things to help enhance your weight loss efforts. First, there are several essential oils that help to suppress the appetite. Next, essential oils can help regulate insulin, which decreases your body's desire to store fats. Also, many essential oils can improve your energy, which makes it easier to stay active. And we all know that moving, exercising, and being active all contribute to weight loss. After all, exercise is an essential component to eight loss. There are even essential oils that can help reduce pain and inflammation, making exercise easier to engage in. There are even some essential oils that help remove toxins from the body and control cravings for certain foods (such as sugary foods), making it easier to keep your desires in check and not feeling deprived when you try to lose weight.

A second thing that many essential oils can do is to improve your mental health. And as we all know, mental and emotional health is a big contributor to weight loss. Most people, if they are stressed, tired, or depressed, start to overeat or eat to help deal with their emotional reactions to things. So, if you are feeling happy, upbeat, and relaxed, you will be less likely to take in these excess calories that make it difficult for people to lose weight. If you feel good, you have more will power and can fight the cravings and desires that you do have.

Using essential oils for weight loss can be done in combination with any diet that you are trying, and that is the beauty of it. Any diet that you decide to follow will be easier to stick to when you add essential oils to the mix. They will help you feel better, more positive, more energetic, help reduce cravings for certain foods and suppress your appetite. And when you feel good and do not feel hungry, you will be able to stick to your diet and lose weight!

This book will first give you all the information you need to know about essential oils in general. The first chapter has a history of essential oils. Here you will learn that plants and their oils have been used for thousands of years, so their voracity has been verified for a very long time.

Chapter two discussed how essential oils can be used specifically for weight loss. It will talk in depth about the specific uses of essential oils to aid in your weight loss journey.

Chapter three will discuss the frequently asked questions about essential oils, their safety, and their use. This chapter will be especially helpful if you have never used essential oils before. It will give you all the information you need to know to get started in using essential oils for weight loss.

Chapter four will discuss the specific oils that are to be used in your weight loss efforts. There are oils that will help with the physical side of losing weight and oils that will assist with the mental and emotional issues that you may encounter while trying to stick with a diet. With this combined approach to weight loss that addresses all of the problems that you may encounter following a diet, you will have a comprehensive plan to weight loss that you can easily stick with. After all, the biggest issues in losing weight are generally emotional eating and suppressing the appetite, and with these two things out of the way, dieting becomes much easier.

The last chapter of the book will discuss mistakes and pitfalls to avoid when using essential oils. If you know what the mistakes and issues are in advance, you can prepare for them, which makes using the oils and losing weight a much easier prospect. After all, you do not need to reinvent the wheel and find them out for yourself. With the knowledge of ages past, you can skip the struggles and get right to the positive outcomes.

When you are done reading this book, you will have all the information you need to use essential oils in a safe and healthy way that will also help you to lose weight. And once you have lost the weight, you can continue to use essential oils to maintain your weight loss. After all, the tools you need to maintain your weight loss are the same ones that you use to lose weight.

Read this book. You will have all the tools necessary to use essential oils to lose weight and to keep it off! So, let's get started on your way to a healthier, happier you!

CHAPTER 1: A BRIEF HISTORY OF ESSENTIAL OILS

An essential oil is defined as a natural oil that is generally obtained through a distillation process of a plant or other source to produce an oil with the characteristic fragrance of that plant. Essential oils have been used for a variety of different purposes all over the world for thousands of years. In fact, the earliest signs of the use of the healing properties of plants were found in France and date as long ago as about 18,000 BCE (20,000 years ago)!

Even our ancestors understood that plants have healing properties that could be used for a wide variety of things.

As for the use of the oils extracted from plants, the earliest evidence that shows their use comes from Egypt in about 4500 BCE. Using these oils was a part of everyday life in Egypt, as they used extracts and oils from plants as medicine, cosmetics, and for medicinal needs. They also used essential oils in their worship services, with each smell being dedicated to each deity. They would then anoint the statues of these gods and goddesses to as part of their worship service and to pay honor to them. However, it did not appear that the Egyptians made their own essential oils. Instead, they imported them from other regions.

China and India are two places that have also used essential oils for thousands of years. China even has written proof of their use of these oils. The Yellow Emperor, Huang Ti, wrote a book called *The Yellow Emperor's Book of Internal Medicine*, which chronicled their uses. Many of the uses of oils in China thousands of years ago are still practiced today. They are truly time-tested. In India, oils were also made into healing potions, with evidence of such acts showing they started about 3000 years ago.

The Father of Modern Medicine, Hypocrites of the Greek civilization, documented the medicinal effects of about 300 plants that are used in essential oils. He got much of his information about these plants from the

Egyptians and the Indians before him. Much of the information can from the exchange of info when Greek soldiers encountered people on the Indian subcontinent while traveling with Alexander the Great.

Hypocrites recommended that people take "a perfumed bath and a scented massage every day is the way to good health." (From his writings). His writings then went on to influence the Romans, with Marcus Aurelius, a Roman emperor, finding a great deal of information about medicine, including essential oils, in the writings.

Once the practice of using essential oils became commonplace in Rome for everyone. Oils and scents were used in baths and massages by regular people and was thought to promote overall health and wellness.

Up to this point, it was the herbs and flowers themselves that were used in the making of the smells, potions, and medicines that were used. It was actually a Persian named Ali-Ibn Sana, who was also known as Avicenna the Arab, who first discovered and wrote down the method for distilling essential oils as we know them today. He was a physician who wrote a book on the properties of about 800 plants, along with their effects on the body. The knowledge he passed down is still in common use today.

During the Crusades, people from Europe learned a

great deal about the Persian methods for distilling essential oils and brought the methods and knowledge back home, where it spread through the European continent. During the 14th century, it was even described how people used Frankincense and pine to ward off the "evil spirits" that they thought were causing the Bubonic Plague. Not surprisingly, documents showed that there were fewer deaths from the plague in places where this practice took place.

Authors from Europe, including Nicholas Culpeper (16753) and chemist Ren-Maurice Gattefosse (1928) wrote about the healing properties of plants and their essential oils. Culpeper's book *The Complete Herbal* and Gattesfosse's book *Aromatherapie*, have both influenced medical practice in Europe and have been transferred to American.

As you can see from this brief history, the healing and medicinal properties of herbs has been knowing for thousands of years and rediscovered by each new generation, with knowledge being spread all over the world. If essential oils did not work, the knowledge of them would have faded into oblivion. However, the exact opposite happened. Because of the healing properties of these plants, more ways to utilize them have becomes known, such as distilling them into essential oils. Then these essential oils are used for a variety of things. The next chapter will talk about the use of essential oils specifically for weight loss. From there, we will discuss all the practical matters you need to know in order to utilize this great tool to help you achieve your weight loss goals.

CHAPTER 2: ESSENTIAL OILS AND WEIGHT LOSS

Essential oils for weight loss are meant to help you approach the difficult task of losing weight in different ways. Because losing weight is both a physical and a mental process, the use of essential oils can help to address both these things. After all, losing weight is more than just about eating less. It is about changing your life, controlling your appetite, dealing with the food cravings that you may have, and handling all the psychological reasons you may struggle with weight loss. If you address all these things, then your journey to weight loss will be much easier.

By using essential oils for weight loss, you can deal with all the areas of your body and mind that you need to deal with in order to lose weight. First, there are the physical needs. Essential oils can help to reduce cellulite, help relieve water retention, and even energizes the body. And, of course, when you feel energized, you are more willing to move and exercise, which adds to your weight loss efforts. Plus, the oils can help you moderate your appetite and reduce cravings for foods that you may desire but sabotage your weight loss efforts.

Next, there are the mental and emotional aspects of losing weight. These are often the ones that most people have some difficulty dealing with. After all, food is more than fuel. Most people nowadays use food to sooth frayed nerves or to make them feel better when they are stressed out, anxious, or depressed. Food has become a source of comfort. This is often one of the reasons that people gain weight and struggle with losing it. When stressed or upset, a pint of ice cream can become dinner, rather than a healthy meal. When bored, instead of finding something to do, we head to the kitchen and check the fridge. We eat mindlessly to make ourselves feel better after the stress of the day. No wonder it is hard to lose weight!

But the beauty of essential oils is that you can use them to deal with not only the physical problems involved in weight loss, you can also use them to help control the mental and emotional aspects! And if you can deal with overcoming your own emotions and mind, then losing weight becomes much easier.

CHAPTER 3: FREQUENTLY ASKED QUESTIONS

This chapter will discuss many of the questions you may have about essential oils, especially if you have never used them before. There seem to be so many options and so much information out there, you may have some difficulty deciding how to use them and how they work. This chapter will discuss all these questions and by the end, you should have all the answers that you need to get started.

How are essential oils used?

There are three methods for using essential oils. They can be applied directly to the skin, inhaled for their fragrance, or in a few cases, ingested. For our purposes, although we will discuss ingesting essential oils in a few cases, this should be done only under the supervision of a licensed healthcare provider. If done wrong, ingesting essential oils can be very dangerous.

To inhale essential oils, there are a few ways to do so. First, you could use a diffuser. The essential oil is placed in a diffuser device (with or without water, read the instructions), which will then heat the scent and put it into the air. It is not recommended that you burn essential oils directly, so this indirect heat method works much better.

The second way that you can inhale an essential oil is through dry evaporation. This only requires wetting a cotton ball with the oil, then leaving it near you, and the scent will diffuse into the air. For a more direct scent, you can sniff the cotton ball.

Third, some people will use steam as an effective way to diffuse the oil. To do this, place one or two drops into a bowl of steaming water. Then, place a towel over your head over the bowl and inhale the steam. Be careful not to use too much of the oil, as this can be a very powerful way to utilize the oils and too much may be overwhelming.

Another way people use to diffuse the smell is to place a few drops of oil in a water-based solution, mixed, and then sprayed into the air. If you prepare an oil this way and keep it around, make sure to shake your spray bottle before each use.

Some essential oils can be ingested. Although most internal uses of these oils should be under the supervision of a licensed health care practitioner, there will be some discussion in this book about the internal use of essential oils. If you choose to follow this use of the oils, make sure that you get 100 percent, pure or food grade essential oils. If you are ingesting oils, you DO NOT want any impurities in your oil. This could cost a little more, but there is no price to your health. We advise that you discuss internal uses with an expert who can guide you properly.

The third way we will talk about using the oils is to apply them topically. This needs to be done very carefully, as the oils can be very powerful and some of them may cause a reaction, especially if you have sensitive skin. It is important to note that most oils need to be diluted to be used in this manner. The general rule of thumb is that the concentration of oil to the carrier substance is no greater than 3 to 5 percent. A carrier substance is what you mix the oil with. This is often water, but can also be a vegetable oil or a nut oil. To get an idea of how much this is, if you use one teaspoon of your carrier (such as water), add one drop of a 3 percent solution. This solution can then be rubbed on the skin.

Other ways to use essential oils include in a bath or as a massage oil. To use in a bath, put a few drops of essential oils into the water right before you step in. If you have sensitive skin, mix the oil with a carrier oil before doing this (see below). Some people also make an Epson salt mixture with essential oils. Mix one part baking soda, two parts Epsom salts, and three parts sea salt. You can then add six drops of the chosen essential oil to the mixture, then add this to the bath.

Also, it can be used as a massage oil. But for this, make sure not to use more than a 1 percent solution of the oil. That means one drop of an oil for every three teaspoons (or one tablespoon) in the oil. It can then be used for massages.

How do I use an essential oil diffuser?

In this book, we will talk a lot about diffusing the scent of an essential oil in a diffuser. There are various types of diffusers available, but they all do the same thing, to allow the vapor from the essential oils you put in them to infiltrate the air around you so that you can reap the benefits of their fragrance. Let's go over the different types of diffusers and how they work.

The first is a candle diffuser. Lit by a candle, there is a reservoir over the flame for the essential oil and water mixture that you are heating. These are simple to use and provide a light fragrance from your oils, but they do not generally produce a strong enough concentration of the scent to provide any real therapeutic benefit. These should be avoided in using essential oils for therapeutic use.

The second type of diffuser is the electric heat diffuser. They work by placing the oil on a small, absorbent pad inside of a heating chamber. This chamber is ventilated, allowing the compound to evaporate in the air. This is a great vehicle for diffusing thicker oils and it requires very little maintenance to use this type of diffuser. However, high heat such as provided in this type of diffuser can damage more volatile essential oils, changing their chemical compound and making them non-therapeutic.

The last type of diffuser available is also the one most people use, and that is the cool air nebulizing diffuser. This system uses air pressure generated by a compressor to vaporize the essential oil in the air. A glass nebulizing bulb serves as the condenser. It gives a strong, therapeutic vapor in the air without relying on heat, so that they compound is not degraded to diffuse it. However, it is also the one type of diffuser that requires regular cleaning, which could become tiresome. Also, certain viscous oils, such as sandalwood oil and ylang ylang oil, cannot be diffused in them. You may need an electric heat diffuser for these.

There is also another kind of diffuser that you can use that will go along with you wherever you go, and it is called diffuser jewelry. There are bracelets, necklaces, and other items that have been designed for putting essential oils in for on the go use. They are like lockets, which open up to reveal a disc that you can then put a couple drops of your preferred oil on to have the scent available to you during the day. It is much easier than carrying essential oils supplies with you.

Where do I buy essential oil supplies?

There are many reputable sellers of essential oil supplies and in many cities and towns. Natural healing clinics, websites, and aromatherapy stores can be located in many places. Just make sure that whoever you buy from is knowledgeable and is selling high-quality items, especially the oils and other ingredients used to make the recipes. This is even more important if the oil you are doing to use is ingested in any way.

What precautions should I take before using essential oils?

Essential oils are very potent, so there are a few things that you should know before using them.

First, do a skin test of the oil. Some people have sensitive skin and may not do well with direct skin contact. If this is the case, use an inhaled method for the oil. Obviously, if you are sensitive to the oil on your skin, do not use it. Second, do not let the oils get into your eyes. Third, make sure to buy the highest quality oils. You do not want to purchase oils with other impurities in it. And if you use an oil and you don't quite feel right afterward, you should discontinue use. You should know whether something makes you feel good or not, and if the answer is no, then you need to discontinue use. Trust your instincts.

And remember, most essential oils should be diluted. Do not use them straight unless the instructions on the oil recommend it. When in doubt, dilute it.

How much of an essential oil should I use?

Less is more when it comes to essential oils. Start

with only a single drop and see what it does. You can always increase a little bit, but if you start with too much, you may have some adverse effects. Other recipes or instructions may dictate otherwise, and you should follow those instructions.

What should I look for when shopping for an essential oil?

Always make sure to get the best quality oils that you can find. If you can, find oils that have not been diluted in any way. Pure oils are best, as long as you know how to properly use them (which we have already discussed). This is because you don't want any unknown additives to your oils that may not be healthy.

Next, make sure that you get oils derived from products that were grown organically. If the plants were grown with pesticides, those will be transferred to the oils. Also, make sure that the oils are tested for purity before being sold. Oftentimes if you cannot find that information on the bottle, it will be listed on the company's website. Knowing that the product has been tested for impurities can be a big relief on the mind.

Getting the best quality essential oils is one of the best things you can do for your health.

What is a carrier oil?

Essential oils are very powerful when used straight up. A carrier oil is a product that is mixed with essential oils to dilute the potent products. Oftentimes water is used, but if the oil is mixed with another oil, that other oil is called a carrier.

There are several different oils that are used as carrier oils. These are some popular carrier oils and the properties they have:

- Grapeseed oil is light and thin and great for massage oils and moisturizing. It has a relatively short shelf life.

- Sweet Almond Oil has a sweet and nutty aroma and is good as an all-purpose carrier oil. Do not use this if you have a nut allergy.

- Jojoba oil has a slightly nutty smell also and has a consistency very similar to the skin's natural oils, making it non-greasy to the touch. It also has a long shelf life.

- Olive oil is easy to find at your local grocery store, but it has a thick, oily consistency, a strong aroma, and a short shelf life. It is popular because you can buy it in any grocery store.

- Fractionated coconut oil is a liquid at room temperature (unlike regular coconut oil) and has no aroma, which makes it better to mix with essential oils because it does not change the fragrance. It does not feel greasy to the touch and has a long shelf life.

- Regular coconut oil is a solid at room temperature and has a coconut odor (unlike the fractionated oil). It, too, has a long shelf life, but it leaves a moisturizing, oily feeling on the skin when applied.
- Shea butter is a solid at room temperature and has a nutty aroma. It is often used as a moisturizer and leaves a waxy feeling on the skin.
- Cocoa butter is a solid at room temperature and many people find it very difficult to work with, so it is less optimal as a carrier oil. Most often, it is used blended with other oils.

Some recipes may call for different carrier oils. These are the most commonly used carriers and something you should keep in your stash.

Should I use essential oils when pregnant or on children?

If you are pregnant, there are some essential oils that you should avoid using. These include basil, cassia, cinnamon bark, clary sage, lemongrass, rosemary, thyme, vetiver, wintergreen, and white fir.

Also, there are things that you should not about essential oil use during pregnancy. First, be very careful during the first trimester. A great deal of fetus development happens during this time, so it is important to be especially careful about how you use essential oils. Second, you should always dilute essential oils if using them when pregnant. Third, if you are unsure, only use oils as an aromatherapy agent and inhale the vapors, as described above. Most of the concern for essential oils comes from topical and internal use of them. If you have any questions, consult an expert in essential oils.

The essential oils that are safe to use while breastfeeding include bergamot, clary sage, grapefruit, geranium, lavender, lemon, melaleuca, patchouli, roman chamomile, sandalwood, wild orange, and ylang ylang. It is also important to note that peppermint can decrease your milk supply, so only use it sparingly while breastfeeding.

As for children, you can use essential oils on them, but it is important to note that you should use them in even more diluted forms than you do for a healthy adult. You should dilute them twice as much as you take them for an adult, and have them only at one-quarter strength for use in babies. Some essential oils can be toxic to children, especially if they are used in high doses. The other thing to note is that you should do when using essential oils on children is to apply them to the bottoms of the feet. Because the skin is thicker there, it will cause less irritation.

What is the difference between aromatherapy oil and an essential oil?

This is a very important question. There is a huge difference between the two, and you need to know. Generally, an aromatherapy oil is a 2 percent strength solution of an essential oil with 98 percent of the solution being either almond or grapeseed oil. The oil and carrier are usually of poor quality and can be very expensive for what you are getting.

On the other hand, an essential oil is undiluted and not mixed with anything. Also, if you are buying a high-quality product, you will not need to worry about any impurities in the oil.

When buying an essential oil, make sure that it is labeled "Pure Essential Oil." If it is labeled anything else, it is not pure. You can also check the company's website to find out about purity testing and quality.

How Should I store My Essential Oils?

There are a couple of things to note when keeping essential oils around, as you want them to stay effective. You want them to be healthy and at their highest potency, so, in order to do so, follow these instructions. First, make sure that they are stored in dark colored bottles since this type of glass will filter out ultra-violet rays from the light that may protect the oils from degradation. Also, never leave your oils out in direct sunlight. Keep them in a cool, dry place. Oils that are exposed to regular, extreme changes in temperature will degrade the oil much faster. To help the oils keep longer, it is best to store in a cool, dark place. If you have room, keep them in your refrigerator. Some oils with carriers may solidify at these cool temperatures, but you can slowly warm up the oil to use it.

Also, it is important to store your carrier oils in the fridge, especially in the summer months, to prevent degradation of the oils. If you cannot store them in the fridge, there are special boxes you can get to store your oils and carriers in to help keep them cool and dark.

It is also very important to keep the oils and carriers away from ignition sources and open flames, as they are moderately volatile and can ignite. They are flammable.

Make sure to tighten the cap on the containers when you are not using them, so they do not evaporate.

Lastly, do not store undiluted oils in plastic bottles. The oils can degrade the bottles and even melt the plastic. Diluted oils in low concentrations can be stored in plastic bottles.

How long can essential oils be stored?

The shelf life of essential oils can vary greatly based on the oil, the storage of it, and other factors. The most important thing that you can do to preserve the effectiveness of an essential oil is to store them appropriately in a cool, dark place, as described above.

If you follow the instructions on storage, most essential oils can be expected to last for two years. The exception to this is that tea tree, pine, and fir oils will last from 12 to 18 months, and cold pressed citrus oils, which will last from 9 to 12 months.

Essential oils do not turn rancid or spoil. Instead, they just lose the therapeutic properties that they contain and chemical chain reactions change the effective ingredients of the oils.

Most carrier oils have a shelf life is 9 to 15 months. Grapeseed oil has the shortest shelf life, lasting only 6 to 9 months. Unlike essential oils, carrier oils do turn rancid. Carrier oils are especially vulnerable to temperature changes, so it is vital that they are stored properly.

The best advice is to buy your essential oil ingredients in smaller amounts so that they are replaced and replenished often. This will solve the problem of whether the oils are still effective.

Now that you have the basic information that you need to get started with working with essential oils, let's dive into the oils needed to work on weight loss. The next chapter will have all the information you need in order to get started losing weight with essential oils!

CHAPTER 4: THE MOST EFFECTIVE ESSENTIAL OILS FOR WEIGHT LOSS AND RECIPES

This chapter will give you the information you need to start losing weight with the use of essential oils. There are three sections. The first section will discuss essential oils that can have an effect on your physical well-being. The second section will discuss essential oils that will help with your mental and emotional well-being. The third section will list other essential oils that you can investigate if needed. You will learn how to deal with stress and other issues that may affect how you view food. If you take this two-pronged approach, you will find great success with your weight loss efforts!

The Physical Side

This section will discuss essential oils that will help deal with the physical problems of weight loss, such as low metabolism, hunger pangs and cravings, and low energy levels. When you improve both of these, it will be easier to lose weight. Speeding up your metabolism enables it to burn more energy, meaning it will burn more fat. This section will also describe oils that help reduce food cravings. With the physical sensations of hunger removed, it is a much easier task to lose weight.

Grapefruit Essential Oil

Grapefruit essential oil has many healing benefits, including the ability to curb food cravings, helping to boost metabolism, helping to increase energy and endurance, and it can even help reduce the accumulation of abdominal fat in the body. It can do all these things because grapefruit oil contains a natural chemical compound called nootkatone, which stimulates an enzyme in the body called AMPK. The interaction between nootkatone and AMPK accelerates chemical reactions in the brain, muscles, and liver, which enables all the benefits listed above. It is also used to help control sugar cravings, so if you have difficulty resisting those donuts in the breakroom or a candy bar, grapefruit oil can do wonders for you. Many people have found great success with weight loss by using grapefruit oil.

There are a couple ways to use grapefruit oil. First, you can use it aromatically by diffusing it through your home in an oil diffuser. You can also inhale directly from a bottle or with the use of a cotton ball, as described earlier.

A simple way to use grapefruit oil topically is to make it into a topical cream. You can do this easily by mixing it into a one to one (1:1) ratio with jojoba oil. You can rub this mixture into sore muscles or on your abdomen to improve digestion.

Also, grapefruit oil is an essential oil that can be used safely internally, as long as the oil you purchase is 100 percent pure, therapeutic grade oil. To ingest this oil, it needs to contain ONLY grapefruit rind oil (the essential oil is derived from the rind). You can add a single drop to a glass of water and drink it or add a drop to honey or a smoothie.

You can also make a cellulite cream out of grapefruit oil. Follow this recipe to do so, then rub it on problem areas to help reduce cellulite buildup.

Total Time: 2 minutes

Serves: 30

Ingredients:
- 30 drops grapefruit essential oil
- 1 cup coconut oil
- glass jar

Directions:
- Mix grapefruit essential oil and coconut oil together. Store in a glass container. Rub into areas of cellulite for 5 minutes daily.
- Make sure to be aware of the adverse effects of any essential oil. Grapefruit oil is considered safe, but it may interact with antidepressants and blood pressure medications. Also, if you are using it topically, stay out of the sun for at least one hour after application. Also, as always, make sure to apply the oil to a small portion of your skin before general use to make sure that you do not have any skin reactions. This is especially true if you have sensitive skin. You should do this with any topical application of any essential oil.

Lemon Essential Oil

Lemon essential oil has properties that can help both with the physical and the emotional aspects of weight loss. It has also been shown to have its properties enhanced when used in conjunction with grapefruit oil. These two oils used together can help with the breakdown of fats in the body, enhancing their weight loss properties.

The effects of lemon oil include suppressing weight gain, increasing energy, enhancing and improving mood, and as a pain reliever. When your mood is improved, people find it easier to stick to their weight loss plan. When negative feelings are dealt with, it is easier to stay positive and have more willpower, especially since many people struggle, more with overeating when they are in a bad mood. And with the physical effects of suppressing the body from storing fat, it has a two-pronged approach to weight loss.

Plus, if pain keeps you from exercising and staying active, lemon oil is a great pain reliever. And with the pain banished from your life, it is easier to establish an exercise routine and stick to it. By taking it after exercise, you can prevent pain from setting in.

To use lemon essential oil for weight loss, you can inhale it off a cotton ball or through a steam bath before you eat. This will help to reduce your appetite, so you eat less without being hungry and are able to lose weight easier. When lemon essential oil vapor is inhaled, it helps to stop you from overeating. Lemon oil, along with peppermint oil (see below), were the two scents that have been proven to prevent overeating and were the most effective in losing weight. These two oils are ones that you need to add to your arsenal!

To make a massage oil from lemon essential oil, add two drops to the carrier oil of your choice and massage it in where fat accumulates. A great carrier oil to use for all weight loss recipes, if not otherwise stated is coconut oil. This helps to eliminate toxins in the fat areas of the body, making them easier to burn.

To use this internally, just add two drops of food grade oil to your morning glass of water to help improve digestion and to eliminate toxins in the body. Again, make sure that your oil is of food grade if you plan on doing this.

To make a spray with lemon essential oil and other oils to spray in your room to promote relaxation, follow this recipe. When you are relaxed and not stressed out, it is easier to stick to your diet and not be tempted to eat to bring up your mood.

Room Spray

Ingredients:
- 6 drops eucalyptus essential oil

- 6 drops bergamot or lemon essential oil
- 4 drops pine essential oil
- 2 drop peppermint essential oil
- 2 ounces purified water

Instructions:

- Combine oils and water in a glass spray bottle. Shake well and spray to combat odors and to promote a relaxing atmosphere.

Peppermint Essential Oil

There are several health benefits to peppermint essential oil, including increasing energy and mental alertness, it improves and elevates the mood, aids in digestion, and helps to reduce appetite. All these effects help you to stick to your diet, as you will be less hungry, food will move through your body faster, and you will have increased energy and mood, leading to a healthier, more active lifestyle without stress-induced eating that so many people suffer from.

Suppressing the appetite is one of the biggest draws of using peppermint essential oil. One study, completed in 2008, showed that people who inhaled peppermint essential oil every two hours reported that they did not feel hungry all the time and ate significantly fewer calories than people who did not inhale the oil. It is worthwhile to use this oil in a diffuser or on a cotton ball to suppress your appetite before every meal. Peppermint oil, along with lemon oil, were the two scents that proved to prevent overeating and were the most effective in losing weight. These two oils are ones that you need to add to your arsenal!

Besides inhaling it, peppermint essential oil is a great one to add to a bath. Add 5 to 10 drops to your morning bath to increase your energy for the day and to help suppress your appetite.

You can also take internally by adding one to two

drops of the food grade, pure oil to reduce appetite and prevent overeating.

Peppermint oil should not as a topical application if you are pregnant or for children under the age of seven.

A good recipe utilizing peppermint oil, grapefruit oil, and lemon oil to help burn fat is to make a capsule from these oils. Use the recipe below to do so. You can buy capsules for essential oil use online or from any good purveyor of essential oils.

Fat-Burning Trio for Internal Use

Have one of these capsules every day after breakfast with a glass of water to help curb your appetite and speed up fat-burning mechanisms. Make sure to buy quality essential oils for internal use (food grade).

Ingredients (per capsule)
- 2 drops peppermint EO

- 2 drops grapefruit EO

- 2 drops lemon EO

- 12 drops coconut oil (liquefied)

Combine the ingredients in one capsule. You could multiply the recipe by mixing the EOs in an amber vial, add six drops of the mix into a capsule together with 12 drops liquefied coconut oil. Store pre-made capsules in the fridge for later use.

Cinnamon Essential Oil

Cinnamon oil has some great properties to help your body avoid weight gain. It improves insulin sensitivity, regulates blood sugar levels, and it reduces inflammation. To understand how it works, you need to understand a little bit about insulin. Insulin works in the body to metabolize carbohydrates and fat, which helps the body absorb blood glucose. It will either convert the carbs and fat to energy or store it. When fat cells in the body no longer respond to insulin, the body starts to store more fat instead of burning it, leading directly to weight gain. This also makes it harder to lose weight. Plus, this is the beginning of Type 2 diabetes. Cinnamon essential oil is used to help improve insulin sensitivity and increase the rate of blood glucose uptake, allowing for easier weight loss.

Cinnamon oil also helps to suppress the appetite and boosts metabolism. Between all these effects, cinnamon is one of the best oils to use for weight loss!

As with the other oils discussed, you can inhale a couple drops on a cotton ball before meals to reduce your appetite. You can also add it to a diffuser to decrease your appetite and make your home smell better.

To take internally, add one to two drops of food-grade cinnamon essential oil to a cup of warm water with a little honey in the morning, before a meal, or at night to avoid craving at night! A couple drops of cinnamon oil can also be added to other recipes to get the same effect. Just make sure that you don't add it to recipes that are cooked at a high temperature, as that can break down the active ingredients.

A good snack to make from cinnamon oil is below. This will help take away the munchies by utilizing cinnamon oil and satisfying that sweet tooth!

Crispy Cinnamon Baked Apple Chips Recipe

Total Time: 1 hour

Serves: 7–8

Ingredients:
- several large organic apples, about 7–8
- 1 tablespoon of your favorite natural sweetener, like raw honey or maple syrup of choice
- 6 drops pure cinnamon essential oil

Directions:
- Preheat oven to 225 degrees F. Line 1–2 baking sheets with some parchment paper greased with coconut oil.
- Thinly slice your apples using a mandolin or knife so they're about the same thickness. Toss the apples with sugar and oil, then add

them to the baking sheet.

- Bake them at no higher than 250 degrees for about one hour, flipping halfway through.

The main concern with cinnamon oil is that it may burn or cause pain when taken internally, especially if you have ulcers in your mouth. Also, this oil could have adverse effects if you have a heart problem, so check with your health care provider if you have any of these issues or you take any medication.

Fennel Essential Oil

Fennel oil is distilled from fennel seeds. It helps to improve digestion, suppresses the appetite, helps prevent the body from gaining more weight, and provides a more restful sleep. And if you sleep better, you are generally in a better mood, which helps curb overeating and emotional eating.

Fennel oil contains melatonin, a hormone that helps to regulate the body's circadian rhythms. In the body, melatonin reduces weight gain by helping the body create more of what is called beige fat, which is known to help burn energy. In the middle ages, fennel was used to help suppress the appetite on religious fasting days. A recent study showed that in laboratory rats, it did help suppress the appetite. Over an eight-week period, rats who inhaled the fennel essential oil twice a day for ten minutes each ate fewer calories and the food passed through the digestive tract faster. Both these things are linked with weight loss.

One way to fight cravings with fennel oil is to put a single drop of it under your tongue to help reduce sugar cravings. This is especially helpful if your weight loss efforts are sabotaged by a sweet tooth.

Inhale fennel seed oil twice a day off of a cotton ball as described previously or through a diffusor to suppress the appetite. The vapors also help you deal with stressful situations, keeping you calm. This will also help in your weight loss efforts.

To make a fennel lotion bar, combine ¼ cup each of coconut oil, almond oil, and beeswax (all carrier oils). Melt these together, then add ten drops each of fennel essential oil and lemon essential oil. Then, pour the mixture into a silicone mold and let it set for 24 hours before using it. This mixture will help keep your skin soft and smooth and is a good way to get the vapors on your body, which will help you suppress the appetite. The combination of the lemon and fennel oils works wonders for appetite suppression.

Emotional and Mental Issues

This section will list essential oils that will help you deal with the mental and emotional sides of weight loss. Depression, stress, anxiety, and general unhappiness will sabotage your weight loss efforts. They cause emotional food cravings, emotional eating, and lessens will power and the desire to stick to the diet as you have chosen. If you deal with these emotions in a healthy and effective way, you will naturally eat less because you won't be driven to make yourself feel better by eating foods that you shouldn't have or that you don't really want.

Bergamot Essential Oil

Bergamot essential oil helps to improve your energy level and boosts your mood. Anxiety and depression are two of the biggest causes of overeating. Of course, overeating will often lead to feeling worse than you did before, even if it gave you some immediate comfort. This starts a vicious cycle that is hard to stop.

But using bergamot oil can stop this vicious cycle. Studies have shown that people who inhale the bergamot oil for fifteen minutes a day reported feeling less stressed and a more positive mood. And we all know that in dieting, feeling good translates into making good food decisions.

To start, inhale the vapors of this oil through a diffuser, steam bath (as described earlier) or on a cotton ball for fifteen minutes a day to improve your mental and emotional health. Many people have reported that this is the perfect oil to inhale in your cranky days to feel better.

Another easy way to utilize bergamot oil is to dilute a few drops in a suitable carrier oil, such as olive oil or coconut oil. Then, use this to massage into your neck or your feet. Doing this in the morning will help to cut down on overeating and will help you deal more productively with negative emotions. You can also add a couple drops of bergamot oil into your morning bath to help you start the day on a positive note and set the tone for a happy day without emotional eating.

Last, the recipe below is a good way to add tension-reducing oils to your bath to help you relax.

Tension Tamer Bath Salt Recipe

Ingredients
- 2 cups Epsom Salt OR Dead Sea Salt
- 1 cup Sea Salt
- 1/2 cup Baking Soda
- 6 drops Bergamot essential oil
- 6 drops Sweet Orange essential oil
- 3 drops Lavender essential oil
- Optional: 6 drops red, 4 drops yellow food coloring

Directions
- Mix salt and baking soda together in a bowl using a metal spoon (a wooden spoon will absorb the essential oils and be ruined.)
- Drop in the essential oils and food coloring, placing each drop in its own little spot on top of the salts. Stir until thoroughly mixed.
- Store mixture in a dark glass or PET plastic jar. Let cure at least 24 hours before using.
- Use about one cup of salts per bath. This bath salt recipe makes enough for three baths.

Be careful with the topical application of bergamot oil, such as in the recipe above, as it can cause sunburn if you are exposed to direct sunlight after application. Also, do not use this oil if you are pregnant. It may cause irritation if you suffer from dry skin. It is also important to note that this is one oil that will degrade very quickly, so only buy it in small amounts that you will use in a short time. Make sure that you store it appropriately, as described above.

Lavender Essential Oil

Lavender essential oil is considered the one of the most essential of oils to use, and has a lot of wonderful effects for becoming more calm and relaxed. It helps to restore the nervous system, promotes sleep, increases inner peace, and helps you deal with panic attacks, anxiety, nervous tension, and even calms a nervous stomach. With all these positive emotional effects, it is one of the go-to oils to use to deal with stress and emotional eating. If you are anxious or depressed, this could be your best solution. Several studies have proven its stress-reducing capacities. If you are an emotional eater or eat when stressed out, you need to add this oil to your arsenal.

We will share with you a couple different recipes to make with the lavender essential oil. Because it is so versatile, it is worthwhile to have it on hand for many different things.

Lavender Bubble Bath

Store this in a bottle and keep it around to relax after a stressful day, instead of reaching for the ice cream!

- 2/3 c liquid glycerin
- 1 c clear, unscented dish soap
- 15+ drops lavender essential oil
- Dried lavender {which will color your bubbles}
- 4 Tbsp. water

- 2 tsp salt

Gently mix in a mixing bowl and add to your container.

The next recipe is for a soothing sleep balm. If you have trouble sleeping, this may serve to help you out. And we all know that we are happier and healthier when we get enough sleep.

Ingredients needed:
- 1/4 cup Lemon balm
- 1/4 cup Chamomile flowers
- Lavender essential oil
- Vitamin e oil
- 1 1/2 cups Coconut oil (You can also use Jojoba oil, olive oil or grapeseed oil)
- 2 Tbsp. Candelilla wax or Beeswax (If using a liquid carrier oil instead, increase wax to 1/4 cup)

Directions:
- Turn your oven on to 200 degrees, then turn it off. Combine coconut oil and herbs in an oven-proof pan/bowl. Stick the herbs & oil in the heated oven. Let them steep for about 3 hours. Use this time to play with your kids. They'll appreciate it.
- Now, take out your herbs and strain the

infused oil into a glass quart jar (or bowl). I really love those mesh strainers that fit into a bowl. You can toss the herbs once they've drained.

- Clean out your pan and pour your strained oil into it. Put it back on the stove and turn it on to low heat. Stir in wax and let it melt. Turn off the heat and add 5 – 10 drops of lavender essential oil. Start low and if it doesn't smell strong enough, add more.

- It's easy to overdo it with lavender, so add a few drops at a time. Then add 10 drops of the vitamin E oil. It helps to keep it from going rancid.

- Pour your balm into dry (make sure they are very dry) jars, put the lid on and wait for it to dry. Make a nice label for your jar(s) so you can remember what's in there.

The third recipe is for an air freshener. To keep lavender in your home and to help keep everyone relaxed, here is a great recipe for an air freshener spray that you can use. The relaxing smell of lavender will keep you calm, relaxed, and away from the comfort food.

What you need:
- 2 cups water
- 1 tbsp. of baking soda
- 15-20 drops of therapeutic grade essential oil

(depending on the strength of the oil you are using)

- You can use just one scent (for example 20 drops of Lavender) or mix scents together (10 drops of Lavender and 10 drops of Chamomile). I prefer using a Lavender/Chamomile blend for bedrooms and a citrus blend of sorts for the kitchen and living room. The possibilities are endless!

Directions:

- Pour the baking soda into a medium sized bowl. Drop the essential oil(s) over the baking soda and mix well. This will ensure that the oil is 'carried' in the powder and does not separate from the water.
- Add the water and stir well until the baking soda has dissolved. Use a funnel and transfer into a spray bottle.
- Spray away knowing that you are filling your home with natural safe scents!

Lastly, here is a simple recipe for a neck rub.

Easy Lavender Neck Rub

Ingredients:

- 3 drops pure lavender oil
- 1 teaspoon fractionated coconut oil or

almond oil

Directions:

- Blend the lavender oil and coconut or almond oil in your palm and rub onto your neck for natural anxiety relief. You can also rub onto the bottoms of your feet. This is perfect for anytime or just before bed.

If you don't have time to make any of the above recipes, you can always just drop two or three drops into your hands or on a cotton ball and inhale the scent when you are feeling stressed and need something to help you relax. If you are having trouble sleeping, rub a drop of lavender essential oil in your hand and then smooth it on your pillow to help you promote good sleep.

Lavender should do wonders for helping you deal with the mental and emotional issues that may cause you to overeat, eat emotionally, or to gain weight. If you have any of these problems, using lavender is an essential tool in your weight loss efforts.

Other Oils to Check Out

The oils listed in this chapter are some of the best and proven oils that you can use to promote the physical, mental, and emotional needs that you have when you are trying to lose weight. However, they are not the only ones that you can use. Once you have investigated some of these oils and incorporated their use in your dieting and weight loss efforts, there are some others you can check out and try.

- Rose oil: This has been shown to be another great essential oil to help relieve depression and anxiety. A ten-minute inhalation and having your feet rubbed with rose oil can do wonders with relieving anxiety.

- Vetiver oils: This oil offers grounding, tranquillity, and reassurance and helps deal with panic attacks. It also helps improve self-awareness.

- Ylang Ylang oil: This oil was featured in one of the earlier recipes. It has been shown to elevate mood, optimism, and to sooth people when they feel fear. It can also help you sleep.

- Essential oils that help to curb appetite: One of the biggest reasons that people fail at losing weight is that they cannot tolerate feeling hungry day after day after day. Some oils to check out for appetite suppression include any citrus oil, juniper, cypress, petitgrain bigarade, and black pepper.

- Other oils to investigate: Tangerine, cloves, spearmint, ginger root, sandalwood, lemongrass, patchouli, celery seed, laurel, eucalyptus, hyssop, rose geranium, and ototea. These oils have been shown to help weight loss efforts in a variety of ways. If you are continuing your weight loss journey and want to add new oils, these are the ones to check out.

CHAPTER 5:
MISTAKES TO AVOID

There are several mistakes that you can make, especially if you are just starting out on your journey with essential oils. This chapter will give you some basic things to watch out for while using essential oils. If you follow these recommendations, your experience with using essential oils will be much more pleasant.

Follow all Safety Recommendations

Just because essential oils are all natural does not mean that they are completely safe. There are recommendations for their use that you should follow, such as:

- Keep oils away from children.

- Do not getting the oils or any products made from the oils in the eyes.

- Do a patch test on a tiny part of your skin to make sure that you are not allergic to an oil or any product you make.

- Take extra precautions if you are pregnant, breastfeeding, or using the oils on children. Check the oils instructions for use in these situations.

- Consult a professional when using oils internally, either a physician or a trained aromatherapist.

- Some essential oils may cause your skin to become phototoxic. Avoid sunlight if you are using these oils topically.

- Make sure to check whether oils may work against each other or cause unwanted side effects when used in combination.

Becoming Desensitized to Oils

If you use then same essential oils over and over, they will start to lose their effectiveness on you. This is because you will become desensitized to their effects. This is why it is a good idea to have a few essential oils that you use for different things. For example, there are a variety of oils listed in this book that will help to suppress the appetite. If one stops working for you, try another. This will help you get the long-term effects that you are looking for.

Mix Oils in the Bath

Essential oils, when added directly to the bathtub, will sit on the top of the water. If you are sensitive to the oils themselves or are using oils with children, mix the essential oil with a carrier oil to prevent sensitivity from bath time use.

Don't Go Cheap

Many people are trying to save money, which is understandable. However, anything that you may put on or in your body should be of the highest quality.

Therefore, it is important that you buy the best oils that money can buy. Make sure that they have been tested and verified pure, and that if you plan on taking them internally, that you get food grade oils only. Make sure the other oils that you buy are therapeutic grade. Buy your oils undiluted and make your own rubs, salts, and other things. If you buy oils that are mixed, you do not know the quality of the oil, and it may not do anything for you.

Ask Questions

It is vital that you ask any questions that you have about using essential oils. This book provides a basic primer, but it may not answer everything that you want to know about. Hooking up with a trained aromatherapist can be one of the best things that you can do. Also, ask suppliers of your products any questions you have about the products you are buying. This may save you spending too much money if you do not buy things that you do not need.

When buying essential oils, there are certain questions to ask, such as:

- Are your oils organic? (Only use organic for therapeutic use.)
- Can you consume these oils?
- Are your oils tested to make sure they are potent and have no additives?

- Are your oils tested by a third party to make sure they do what you say they will?
- Do you visit the farms where the plants are grown for your oils? Are you sure of their sustainability and voracity?

Learn As Much As You Can

This book is a great start for using essential oils to help you lose weight, but you may be interested in incorporating more essential oils into your life. Take a class, get more books, and talk to people trained in the use of essential oils. It is a deep subject with many opportunities for learning. This book gives you the basics that you need to start, but there is so much more information out there. Don't be afraid to explore the field.

Make Sure to Handle Your Oils Correctly

Some people new to essential oils don't treat the oils with the respect that they need. In an earlier chapter, we discussed how to handle and store your oils. If you do not follow these guidelines, your oils will not retain their therapeutic effects. Many people choose to buy their oils in small amounts to avoid them losing their potency. Follow the storage recommendations in the FAQ section for the best outcome after storing oils.

Do Not Put Oils Everywhere On Your Body

If an oil can be used on the body, they are normally specified as to where to use it and how often. Oils should not be out all over your body. Also, be aware of whether the oils will make you more susceptible to sunburn.

You CAN Overdose on Essential Oils

Make sure to always use the oils as directed. Too much use of an oil can lead to overdose. Remember, even natural products have specific directions for use. The recommendations in this book for the specific oils used for weight loss and the information on the bottles that you will buy should be followed. Failure to do so could cause several problems.

Don't Give Up

If one essential oil does not work for you, try another. Just like medications, not all oils will work exactly the same way for all people. The concept of bio-individuality is at play here, meaning that what works for someone else may not work for you. As we have stated earlier, there are several different oils that may have the same effects, so it is worth experimenting and seeing what works best for you.

CONCLUSION

Hopefully by now you have learned all you need to know in order to utilize essential oils for weight loss. By now, you have the information you need to use and store essential oils safely, the recipes and techniques that you should implement the oils in everyday use, and what to look out for. Plus, once you have lost the weight you desire, you can continue to use these techniques to maintain your weight loss. Essential oils are something that you can incorporate into your life for the rest of your life.

Good luck on the journey!

You may also like these books

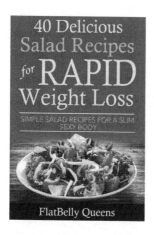

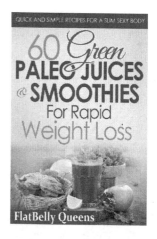

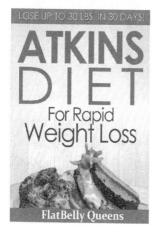

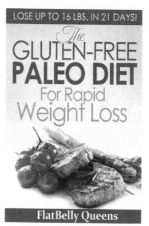

Made in the USA
Lexington, KY
13 September 2017